The Silent Flute

A Walk in the Footsteps of Alzheimer's Disease

By Todd J. Hubley

authorHOUSE®

AuthorHouse™
1663 Liberty Drive
Bloomington, IN 47403
www.authorhouse.com
Phone: 1-800-839-8640

First published by AuthorHouse 6/24/2009

ISBN: 978-1-4389-8131-4 (sc)
ISBN: 978-1-4389-8132-1 (hc)

Printed in the United States of America
Bloomington, Indiana

This book is printed on acid-free paper.

Special Thanks

This project began as a short film to be titled 'The Wisdom of the Aged'. Through the process of many interviews and conversations it has become what it is today; The Silent Flute. I have so many people to thank for their inspiration and help with this work. From everybody who ever shared a story or a comment or an encouraging word to the people listed here, I thank you all.

First and foremost I owe a heartfelt thank you to Professor Al Jacobs. Al and I spent many hours working together in Menlo Park and Sausalito on the plot lines and stories. Without his passion for film and willingness to guide me, this project would have stalled on the starting line. I thank you Al.

I must also thank Marjorie Smith. Ms. Smith retired from her career as a school principal more than 30 years ago and after a few hours of interviews it was clear that the people of her generation certainly do have stories to share. Sharp as a tack at nearly 90 years old Marjorie offered no insight into the world of Alzheimer's disease, she did however; inspire the original foundation of 'The Wisdom of the Aged'. I thank you Marjorie.

For more reasons that just this book I thank my mother Michele Hubley and Aunt Laura Paparatto. These two lovely ladies gave the work a voice. Michele helped me to envision the film and hear the music. Laura literally recorded the music and brought a piece of the project into the real world with her flute. I thank you both; Laura and Michele.

I would also like to thank my wife Yoko Hubley for providing me with endless support and understanding. A friend once asked me how Yoko could possibly put up with me – "she must be an angel!" he said. He was right. I thank you Yoko.

Contents

Chapter 1
A Fond Farewell
Spring 2001

Kathryn Wilder takes a deep breath of the crisp, clean air of spring that has enveloped the island of Manhattan. Around her, New Yorkers are bustling about with that rare positive energy that seems to flow throughout the city. People are no longer bundled up in their winter clothes. Instead, they wear light layers, reflecting the new season as they walk with a renewed bounce in their steps.

Everything about today seems to signify a new beginning. Everything, that is, except the event she and her five-year-old son, Bobby, are getting ready to attend. Her father, the professional flute player Jonathon Rayne, is giving his farewell performance at Radio City Music Hall.

A throng of people is milling about outside Radio City. A buzz is in the air as people chat and smoke their last cigarettes before going inside to take their seats. Kathryn and Bobby make their way through the crowd and are quickly escorted to their seats at the front of the auditorium. Although they have backstage passes hanging around their necks, they are well aware that Jonathon, whom they affectionately refer to as Grandpa, prefers to prepare for the show alone. They'll go back to congratulate him after the show ends.

Kathryn is a bit disappointed because Rob, her husband, has just called to inform her that he has to work late. He was supposed to meet them in front of Radio City before the show. Still, this night belongs to her father, and she feels so much excitement and pride for him and all of his accomplishments. The lights dim, and Kathryn watches as

Bobby leans forward in his seat, wide-eyed with excitement to see his grandfather playing in front of all these people.

As the curtain opens, Jonathon Rayne appears. He's wearing a tuxedo and is holding a golden flute. Accompanied by a piano and a harp, Jonathon begins to play. Kathryn is speechless as the sweet melody captivates the audience. Bobby sits up in his seat. His eyes are wide and his mouth is open, and he seems completely mesmerized by the grandeur of his grandfather's playing. Of course, Kathryn and Bobby have heard Grandpa play a thousand times before, but it's never been like this. This is his final show, and the emotions are running high.

If Kathryn did have one wish for tonight it would be that her mother, Laura Jean Rayne, were alive to see this show. Still, Kathryn knows that her mother is at this very moment looking down over them with a smile on her face, perhaps even playing along with her husband!

The music is magical in a familiar way to Kathryn. Although she is quite captivated by her father's playing, her mind cannot help but wander. She daydreams of all the good times past. There was a time when she was much younger that her father brought her up on stage at his shows. She smiles to herself just thinking about how normal that felt, how unafraid she was. Back then her mother was the piano accompanist. The family was very close, and her parents always included her in their professional lives. Still, she is grateful that they never pressured her to pursue a career in show business.

Her mind returns to the moment as the final selection reaches its crescendo. The audience erupts in applause. Grandpa lowers his flute and smiles as he enjoys the accolades.

"Thank you all very much. Thank you," he says.

He then motions his arms to settle the crowd. The entire auditorium falls silent. Jonathon speaks to his adoring fans for the last time.

"Thank you. Wow, what a great night. Thank you all for coming. This is my last piece, and I want to dedicate it to my daughter, Kathryn, and to my grandson, Bobby."

Grandpa gestures to Kathryn and Bobby in the front row as he says these words. The smile on Bobby's face manages to get even bigger and brighter, reflecting the pride he feels in his grandfather. And he is clearly very happy to have had his name mentioned in front of all these people.

As if the three of them were the only people in the room, Grandpa says, "Kathryn, Bobby, thank you for coming tonight."

Grandpa begins playing his final encore, "Meditation from Thais" by Jules Massenet. The listeners are transfixed on him and enchanted by how beautifully he is playing. Even Kathryn, who has heard him play this piece a thousand times, is drawn in and captivated by the music.

Grandpa reaches the crescendo, and as the final note is being played, the audience members begin to applaud. They rise, and a long, heartfelt standing ovation ensues. Kathryn and Bobby stand and clap as loud and enthusiastically as they possibly can.

The curtain closes for the final time, and lights are turned up. As the auditorium begins to empty, Kathryn and Bobby make their way backstage where they are told to wait while Grandpa changes his clothes. As soon as they are given the okay, Bobby bursts through the door and runs toward his grandfather, who is sitting on a chair tying his shoes.

"Grandpa! Grandpa!" Bobby yells. "You were great!"

Grandpa lifts Bobby onto his knee. "Not too shabby for an old man, eh?" he says.

"When I grow up I want to play here with you, Grandpa," Bobby says as he hugs his grandfather.

"You got it, Bobby!" Jonathon says. "What about you, Kathryn? What did you think?"

"Dad, you were magnificent!" she tells her father. "I can't remember ever hearing you play so well."

"What did you think of the encore?" he says. "You know, I don't know if I ever told you this, but your mother—your grandmother," he says looking at Bobby, "and I used to play that together in Vienna right after we met."

"Did my grandmother play the flute too?" Bobby asks.

"Oh, no, Bobby. Your grandma was a majestic pianist. We were a great duo. I only wish she were alive to enjoy this moment."

"Hey, Mommy can play the piano too, you know!"

"Oh yes, I know," he says as he winks at his daughter. "Maybe when you get older we can persuade her to play here with us."

"Oh, no you don't!" Kathryn retorts. "I'm not nearly good enough, and besides, the thought of being in front of all of those people scares me half to death."

Grandpa smiles and lifts Bobby off of his knee as he stands up.

"You didn't used to be frightened," he says with a smile. "Hey, what happened to Rob? Wasn't he supposed to meet you here?"

"Yes, but you know Rob, always working. He called me on the cell phone just before the show. He should be at home by the time we get there."

"I don't know how he does it," Grandpa says while shaking his head. "Come on, Bobby, let's get outta here. Maybe we can get some ice cream on the way home, huh?"

"Yeah! Ice cream!" Bobby hollers as he skips down the hall.

Chapter 2
Three Generations in Music
Spring 2003

Kathryn has been working hard for the past couple of years since her father's concert at Radio City Music Hall. She works for Y&A Inc., which produces and distributes instructional DVDs, offering lessons in everything from algebra to zoology. The company and industry are a perfect fit for Kathryn because they allow her to combine her creative talent with her technical interests.

In fact, Kathryn was recently promoted and now heads up the arts and music division. Of course, she has to be business savvy to lead the division, but her real passion comes out when she is working closely with the engineers and artists in the studio during productions. Although Kathryn's musical prowess probably could have led to a life in show business, she wanted to live a more stable lifestyle in order to raise a family. She grew up on the road, and she didn't want that for her children.

On the other hand, her husband's job demands a significant amount of traveling. Rob is an account executive for a computer systems company called Serten. The company makes and installs multimillion-dollar billing systems that integrate consumer billing across various lines of business.

Rob's job is business development and sales, which includes oversight and follow-up after the systems are installed. Because he is the main contact for his customers until the systems are fully integrated, his time is not his own. He is generally on call for two to three projects running simultaneously. After the system is up and running, the client is serviced exclusively by the technical support team.

With two working parents and the amount of traveling required of Rob, Kathryn was concerned that Bobby wouldn't get to experience the rewards of a close-knit family. So about a year ago, Rob and Kathryn, along with input from Bobby, asked Grandpa to move in with them, and he accepted. Kathryn was sure her father based his decision in part on his loneliness, but mostly on the idea that he would get to spend a lot of time with his grandson.

At the time, Grandpa lived in a small house in Sparta, Connecticut, about five miles from the Wilder family home. They all loved the little town; it afforded them the lifestyle of the suburbs and the convenience of being just over an hour from New York City. They found a five-bedroom home on a nice street in the same school district that Bobby was attending.

Now that the family has lived together for about a year, they have a working routine and new family dynamic. As Kathryn is finishing the dishes one night in May, Rob sits at the kitchen table watching Bobby practice his puppet show for school. Kathryn can hear her father playing his flute in the music room.

As Bobby manipulates his puppets from behind a stage made out of boxes, the sound of the flute stops. Kathryn turns on the faucet as Grandpa walks into the kitchen with a photograph in one hand and his flute in the other. He says something to her, but she can't hear a word over the sound of the running water.

"Dad," Rob says, "where is the newspaper?"

Her father looks annoyed at the question as he points across the room and says curtly, "Where I always put it— over there on the counter."

Rob gets up from his chair and retrieves the newspaper off the counter. He sits back down and removes a pen from his shirt pocket. He flips open the paper and proceeds to do the crossword puzzle. Rob has taken to doing the crossword puzzles fairly regularly. However, Kathryn knows he doesn't have the patience to think through those kinds of puzzles. Generally, he ends up questioning the family for most of the answers. Still, it doesn't stop him from trying, and it sure doesn't stop him from looking proud and taking all the credit—which she is glad to give him—when they are complete.

Now that she has finished with the dishes and can better hear, Grandpa again addresses Kathryn.

"Did your people reserve the studio yet?" he asks.

"Yup," she says as she dries her hands with a dish towel.

"We're all confirmed for the last week in August. You're sure there's enough time between now and then for you?" she asks.

"Absolutely, that's plenty of time. I've finished with the composition; I just need to polish it up. Three months should be more than sufficient," he replies.

Kathryn knows that behind the makeshift puppet stage, Bobby has been listening to the conversation between her and his idol, Grandpa. Bobby's puppet show is supposed to include a new piece of music composed by Grandpa, and the project is due next week. Bobby has told his mother that he's worried that the piece might not be ready in time. Grandpa has been crediting Bobby with helping him to write the piece, although in all honesty, Bobby more or less just asks a lot of questions. Still, both of them seem to have enjoyed the time they've spent "working" together. But Kathryn realizes that now Bobby is concerned with what his grandfather is saying, especially when he begins using the puppet to talk to Grandpa.

"Three months is too long. Bobby has to do the puppet show next week. And besides that's what Grandpa and me—I mean Bobby—wrote it for."

"That's exactly right," Grandpa says to the puppet, "and Bobby and I are going to record it together here this weekend. His mommy and I are just talking about recording it again later for her company. We're going to put it on a DVD."

Bobby looks satisfied with his grandfather's explanation. "Okay," he says. He lowers the puppet off the stage and starts to flip pages in his script, apparently trying to figure out a good starting point to resume his rehearsal.

Kathryn turns her attention back to her father and notices the picture in his hand. She tilts her head to get a better look at it.

"Dad, is that the picture you were talking about for the insert?" she asks.

Her father doesn't answer. Instead, he seems lost in the photograph.

"Dad?" she asks again.

"Huh? … Oh, yes, yeah, it is."

"That's you and Mom in Vienna, before you were married, right?" Kathryn asks. Her father responds with a simple nod of his head.

As usual, Rob is oblivious to the family's actions and conversations as he diligently works on his crossword puzzle. Now he interrupts to say, "I need a six-letter word for a nineteenth-century composer, beginning with the letter 'C'."

Grandpa gives it a moment's thought. "Tchaikovsky," he finally says.

"No! Six letters," Rob says. "And anyway, doesn't Tchaikovsky begin with a 'T'?"

Grandpa seems a little bit embarrassed, but he continues to try to come up with the answer. He even counts the letters of a name on his fingers. Finally, he looks satisfied. "Brahms," he says emphatically.

"No! It has to begin with a 'C'," Rob says sounding annoyed.

At that, Bobby's voice comes from behind the box stage. "Chopin!"

Kathryn is quite surprised that her father is unable to come up with the right answer. She half looks at her father as she congratulates Bobby for getting the correct answer.

Grandpa, who is equally surprised, simply says, "I knew that. I was just kidding."

Chapter 3
The Recording Studio
Summer 2003

The New York offices of Y&A have a series of studios for video and music production. Today, music Studio B has a handwritten sign posted on the door that reads, "Three Generations of Music." Kathryn has reserved the studio so they can record the finishing touches for the DVD.

Dan Gray, the project's producer, has worked with Jonathon Rayne many times throughout the years. He produced almost every record and album that Jonathon recorded. Like her father, Dan retired a couple of years ago. However, Kathryn has been able to talk him into working on a few projects for her company from time to time.

Inside the studio, Kathryn and Dan are making the last-minute preparations for what should be the final day of recording. Kathryn can't help but think back on what it has taken to get here. She knows that her father wrote the new composition with his whole family in mind. He even insisted that both Kathryn and Bobby be involved in the different aspects of the educational DVD.

In the course of many years of conversations, Kathryn and her father came up with a vision to create a learning tool for up-and-coming musicians. With Kathryn leading the behind-the-scenes production and technical aspects of the project, Bobby would play the role of the emerging protégé, and his grandfather, the renowned flute player, would instruct him on intermediate music theory and the finer points of performing in front of an audience.

At this point, all of the heavy lifting is done; the crews have finished filming and editing, so all that remains are the finishing touches on the soundtrack. Kathryn has the studio only for the time she'd reserved months before, and she, Dan, and Grandpa have already used up a few days. Time is running out, and the process seems to be moving very slowly.

The studio is a remarkable place to work. The medium-sized soundproof room contains a microphone, headsets, a PA system, and a comfortable padded stool. A spit shield is attached to the front of the microphone to reduce the sound of Grandpa's breath as he blows across the flute's mouthpiece. Grandpa is sitting in this soundproof room rehearsing.

Kathryn and Dan are on the other side of a big glass window working out the details of the day. Their room is equipped with a high-tech mixing board, speakers, and monitors. This is where they sit while recording music and lyrics and editing.

"Do you think he'll be okay today?" Dan asks as he and Kathryn finish up the day's goals.

"He's fine," she says. "He was just nervous yesterday. He hasn't recorded professionally in a long time. There's no problem, Dan, really."

"Come on, Kathryn. You know as well as I do that it's not just what happened yesterday. He's been screwing up a lot, even during the rehearsals. I've known your father for a long time. It's not like him."

"Dan, I said there's not a problem," Kathryn says emphatically. "I spoke with him last night. He's fine."

"Well, let's hope so, 'cause if he isn't we're going to be out a whole lot of money."

"Let's just get started, all right?"

"You're the boss!"

Kathryn walks over to the door that leads to the room where Grandpa is supposed to be practicing. As she opens the door, she sees her father sitting on the stool in front of the microphone. However, he is not practicing his flute; instead, he is reciting something as if he were in front of a huge crowd.

"… Yet knowing how way leads on to way," he says, "I doubted if I should ever come back. I shall be telling this with a sigh, somewhere ages and ages hence: two roads diverged in a wood, and I—I took the one less traveled by, and that has made all the difference."

"Robert Frost?" Kathryn guesses.

Her father seems startled at her interruption. He looks up at her, not embarrassed or guilty, but just gives her a look.

Then, in a more inquisitive tone and not answering her, he asks, "Yes?"

"We're ready when you are, Dad."

Kathryn closes the door and walks over to stand behind the glass window. Dan shoots her a nervous glance. The tape starts to roll, and they are recording. Grandpa just sits on the stool with his flute in his hand and stares at Kathryn. It's as if he doesn't even know who she is. Kathryn motions to her father to put the flute to his lips.

When he finally does press his lips to the mouthpiece, he begins to blow. But it's as if he can't even make a sound with the instrument. He looks frustrated, as if he knows that he can play the flute. But more than frustrated, he looks frightened. And that look is enough to know that there is something seriously wrong with Grandpa.

Chapter 4
Who Is Tommy?
Winter 2003

One room in the family's house is entirely devoted to Grandpa's music. It's not entirely soundproof, but the walls are insulated to muffle any noise coming from or going into the room. Kathryn knows that her father thinks of the room as a sort of sanctuary and loves being in there, whether or not he's working.

The rest of the family refers to it as "the Music Room." It is basically a shrine to Jonathon Rayne's career, with old concert posters and performance photographs hanging on the walls. Jonathon has a lot of memorabilia and photographs from the different venues he's played. Even more impressive is the number of different artists with whom he's worked. This is also the room with the most pictures of Kathryn's mother, looking so young and beautiful.

Bobby is in the Music Room playing Monopoly with his grandfather when Kathryn walks in carrying a bowl of peas.

"Who didn't eat their peas?" she asks angrily.

"I ate mine," Bobby answers quickly. "It was Grandpa; I saw, he didn't eat his."

"Why are you always trying to get me into trouble, Tommy?" Grandpa complains.

Kathryn walks over to her father and hands him the bowl of peas and a spoon. She tells him, as she has many times before, that he must eat his peas for the nutrition. He looks completely put out by her demand because he doesn't like peas. He simply takes the bowl from her without responding.

"Mom," Bobby says as he follows his mother toward the door. "How come Grandpa keeps calling me Tommy?"

"Tommy was Grandpa's brother. He died a long time ago—even before you were born."

"But why is he calling me Tommy?" Bobby asks as they stop at the doorway.

"Well, we need to talk about that. Grandpa is sick."

Meanwhile, Grandpa is unaware of the conversation taking place on the other side of the room. He is holding the bowl of peas and poking at them with his fingers.

"What's wrong with him?" Bobby asks.

"He has what's called Alzheimer's disease."

"Old timer's disease. What's that?"

"Not 'old timer's'" says Kathryn. "Alz-hi-mers. It just means that he gets very forgetful, and sometimes he doesn't seem like Grandpa. But never think that he doesn't still love you—he does. He loves you very much."

Suddenly, peas begin to fly across the room. Grandpa is shooting them around the room with his spoon. He's putting a couple of peas on the spoon, holding the end of the handle with his right hand, and pulling back the other end, sending the peas flying as they would from a catapult. Peas are hitting the walls, concert posters, and pictures.

"Dad! What in God's name do you think you're doing?" Kathryn yells almost hysterically. "Stop that right now. I told you to eat those ..."

"I don't want these fucking—these fucking—green things, goddamn it!" he yells back. Kathryn is stunned by her father's use of the word "fuck."

"Dad! First of all, I don't want you using that kind of language, especially around Bobby. And secondly, it's not a choice. You have to eat those peas."

Grandpa, boiling over with anger, hurls the bowl across the room and into the wall. "No, no, no!" he yells as the bowl smashes and peas fly everywhere.

Kathryn is now more scared than she is angry. She is scared of the potential danger that her father poses to Bobby. Grandpa sits down at the desk in the corner of the room and is seemingly oblivious to what has just transpired.

"Bobby, go on up to your room," Kathryn says.

"Mom, what's happening?"

"I'll be up in a minute, but right now I need you to go upstairs to your room."

As Bobby leaves, Kathryn isn't sure what to make of the situation. Her father seems to be calm and nonthreatening now. He twists back and forth in his chair as she starts to pick the peas up off of the floor.

"Dad, you could've hurt somebody. What's gotten into you? Huh? What is going through your head that would make you do that?"

"Can I have a banana?" he asks simply.

Kathryn looks at her father in disbelief. Confused and defeated she says, "Sure," and leaves the room to go get the banana.

Chapter 5
Kathryn Seeks Support
Summer 2004

A few months ago Kathryn made the decision to quit her job so that she could care for her father fulltime. Although she knew that it would be difficult, she wasn't really prepared for the emotional rollercoaster ride that would ensue. Each day brings with it a different challenge; her father may be difficult, unruly, and absentminded, or he may be the fun-loving and talented father Kathryn has always known.

At the recommendation of her father's doctor, Kathryn decides to try out a support group for the primary caregivers of Alzheimer's patients. She knows the troubles that she has been facing, and she thinks it may be a good idea to commiserate with others.

Rob does listen to her and he sympathizes, but he doesn't really understand what she goes through on a daily basis. He has to go to work, which involves some traveling. So even if he would like to help more, it's impossible for him to do so. Still, more important than airing out her own issues, Kathryn wants to hear what other people in her situation are going through.

Kathryn called Dr. Rivers, the woman who runs the group, and asked if she could join. It had been surprisingly easy. There was no initial visit or large expense associated with the meeting. In fact, Dr. Rivers, who asked to be called Kathy, invited Kathryn to the group's next meeting.

Kathy explains that the group meets once a month for an hour or so. "It's not really therapy," she says. "I'm more like a conductor than a psychologist. We're not trying to cure anybody or bring out demons, so to speak. It's really just to bring people together who in some way are each affected by Alzheimer's."

As she walks into the meeting room for the first time, Kathryn is surprised to see only five other people in the group. She takes a seat in the circle as the meeting begins. "Good evening, everybody," says Dr. Rivers. "As you all know, I'm Kathy, and I started this support group while dealing with my father's battle with Alzheimer's. Since his death, I still find it very therapeutic to work though the challenges with others. I'd like to welcome our new members, Melissa and Kathryn. Melissa, let's start with you. You said your mother is getting worse. Why do you feel that way?"

"Well, she does have her good days," Melissa says. "But you know, those days are really when she's remembering and realizing that she has bad days. So it's almost as if her bad days are better for her than her good days. I don't know if that makes any sense."

"It makes a lot of sense," says Chris, a man in his sixties. "And that's something that has taken me a long time to realize, a lot longer than it seems to have taken you. But I think it's true; their good days can actually be painful and frightening to them. I know, at least with my sister, she would get all in a condition when she would see something or realize something, and it would hit her that she should know what it meant. She'd end up getting very confused and frustrated because she realized that she didn't. And honestly, I think that I only made things worse for her by pushing her to understand. You know, saying things like, 'It's me, Chris, your brother. Remember me?'"

"That's it exactly, Chris!" says Melissa. "Sometimes I feel like I should play along, and other times I think I should try and help my mother understand. The thing is, I don't know when to do what.

"The other day I was staying at my mom's, and I heard her screaming," Melissa says. "Not like a bloodcurdling scream, more like a cry for help. Anyway, when I got up to her room, she was sitting up in bed and pointing to the floor, saying, 'The child has fallen through the hole,' and she cautioned me to be careful around the hole. I have no idea what she was talking about, so I just sort of played along and told her that I would be very careful."

"You know, sometimes they really are like kids in a way," says Michele, a woman of about forty. "My mother has Alzheimer's, and it's often like having another child in the house. Kids let their imaginations run wild, often to the point where they almost see the spaceship or army fort that they have created. It seems to be the same sort of thing with my mother, only I can't rationalize with her to stop. I mean, I can tell a child to stop fooling around, but an Alzheimer's patient cannot rationalize in that way. If they see a hole in the floor—whether it's a shadow or because they have cataracts—then, to them, there is a hole in the floor."

"Very nicely put, Michele," complimented Dr. Rivers. "One thing that you can try, Melissa, is to bring her over to where she thinks the hole is. Take her by the hand, reassure her that everything is okay and that she is safe, and then let her touch the floor. Of course, the next day she may well see the hole again, but it may help to calm her in the moment if she is really frantic about it."

"My mother is in the late stages of the disease," says Sandy, a woman in her thirties, "and my father died not too long ago, after taking care of her for years. Anyway, for those of you who don't know, my mother is Japanese, born and raised in Tokyo, and my father was an American. If Alzheimer's isn't painful enough, making my poor father unrecognizable to his wife, she deteriorated to the point where often they couldn't communicate because my mother was left without an understanding of the English language."

"Do you speak Japanese?" Kathryn asks.

"My father regretfully didn't, but I do," Sandy replies. "And at times my mom can speak English again. It's strange, and sometimes it can even be funny. A couple of weeks ago I was in my mom's kitchen making tea when she walked in. I looked over at her, and with a puzzled look on her face, she said, 'I don't know who you are, but I know you're not George.' George was my father, and it's a bittersweet moment because I know that my father must have been smiling down on us!"

Chapter 6
What's Going on in There?
Autumn 2004

Rob is sitting in the living room reading the morning paper and drinking a cup of coffee. He is already dressed in a suit and ready to leave for work. Kathryn hates interrupting his morning activities, but she's worried about her father.

"Rob," she says as she approaches the living room.

"What?" he asks without looking up from the paper.

"Rob, I'm really worried about what's going on in there."

"In where?" he says impatiently as he lowers the paper. "What are you talking about?"

"He went into the bathroom, same as every morning, but I don't hear any water. What could he be doing?"

"I don't know; using the toilet maybe, clipping his toenails," Rob says sarcastically. "There are about a million things he could be doing in there. Just let the man be; he's fine."

"Rob, he's been in there for half an hour. Please go up there and check on him."

"Why don't you just knock on the door, Kathryn?"

"I don't want to embarrass him."

"Oh, but it's okay for me to?"

She knows that Rob realizes that no matter what logical thing he says, nothing is going to change her mind. He will end up going upstairs to see what her father is doing in the bathroom. Finally he stands up, puts his paper down on the chair, and heads that way.

"Just peak in," Kathryn says as they reach the bathroom door.

"Oh sure, that won't embarrass the poor guy. I can see it now. 'Sorry, Dad, just wanted to make sure you didn't fall in!'" Rob says with a bit of a laugh.

"Stop it. Just knock on the door, and if he doesn't answer, just peak in."

"Okay, okay."

Rob presses his ear against the bathroom door and listens. "You're right," he says. "I don't hear any water running. It's almost completely silent in there." He then knocks ever so softly on the door. "Dad?" he whispers. "You in there? Dad?"

"Open the door," Kathryn says impatiently.

Rob seems irritated by her request as he turns around and looks at her. Still, she thinks he knows not to push her buttons right now. So he opens the door just enough to poke his head into the room and then turns around with a smile on his face.

"You have to see this," he says to Kathryn.

"What? Is everything all right?" she asks as she steps up to the door and looks inside.

"Well, why does he even bother to get up and go in there?" she asks when she sees her father in his pajamas, fast asleep while sitting on the toilet.

"I don't know, but it doesn't look like he needed to be in there at all," Rob says with a chuckle.

"I guess that explains why it seemed like he wasn't bathing. He's not. He must be getting up in the morning and going into the bathroom out of habit. The good news is that he knows he's supposed to go in there, but the bad news is that he doesn't seem to know why," she says.

"Actually you're right, and we'll need to fix that. Why don't you ask at your group what we should do to get him to take a shower?"

"I'll add that to the list."

Chapter 7
Labeling
Early 2005

Kathryn returns from the grocery store to find labels on all of the kitchen cabinets and drawers. As she puts the groceries away, she is mystified and incredulous. She's not sure what to make of the effort. She leaves the kitchen and heads for her bedroom, where she presumes Rob is.

When she gets to the room, sure enough, he is there and is putting his label printer back on the closet shelf. She notices several books dealing with the topics of senile dementia and Alzheimer's disease.

"Did you see what I did in the kitchen?" Rob says proudly.

"I did," Kathryn replies, "and thank you, but it really wasn't worth the trouble."

"No, no, I'm glad to help. In fact, I keep—"

"Thing about it is, Rob," Kathryn interrupts, "it's not going to help. My father's not a child; we can't teach him. This disease is degenerative. He's just going to get worse and worse."

"Well, what if we draw pictures and put those up on the cabinets?"

"Rob, you're not listening to me. It's too late for labels. He's past that point. And he can't conceptualize in that way now."

"What the hell are you talking about?" Rob asks angrily. "Are you telling me that if I put a picture of a loaf of bread on the bread box, your father won't know that there is bread in there?"

"That is precisely what I'm telling you. Maybe if you had thought of it six months ago, it would have helped, but now it's too late. His mind doesn't make the connections anymore. There's nothing we can do to bring that back. It's gone—forever."

"So ... what, what can I do?" Rob asks, looking confused and a bit stunned. "Where does that leave us?"

"I don't know, Rob. I just don't know," says Kathryn. Then, after a pause and with a nervous giggle, Kathryn adds, "I do know that this disease could be genetic, so maybe you should keep the kitchen labeled for me."

"Oh, come on, Kathryn. You're being ridiculous."

"Am I? Am I, Rob?" she says while picking up a couple of the Alzheimer's books. "I've read all there is to read about this disease, and so far the descriptions and my father's actions have been dead-on. Think about it; our biggest problem used to be that when he said he was looking for a needle, he really wanted a comb. Now ..."

"It's not that bad. We can deal with it."

"We?" Kathryn retorts. "Jesus Christ, Rob, you're not here with him all day. I am. When he gets up, he has no idea who I am. I then spend most of the day fighting with him to eat, take pills, or bathe. The simplest actions take hours. He lashes out every single time something is uncomfortable or confusing."

"Well then, we'll just have to be more strict with him," says Rob.

"You're not listening," Kathryn yells. "He's not a child, and I sure as hell can't control him physically. He's strong, and when he decides he doesn't want something, I can't force him."

"What do you want from me, Kathryn?" Rob shouts back. "I'm sorry I can't be here twenty-four hours a day; someone has to work to put food on the goddamn table. I don't have the answers. You've 'read all there is to read about this disease.' So, you tell me, what do those books say to do?"

Kathryn stares at her husband. She knows she isn't being fair to him, but that's not her biggest concern as he leaves the room in a huff. He has raised a good point about the books, and it is becoming clear what she has to do. It's a big decision, and she's been in denial about how serious the situation is becoming.

Kathryn, feeling defeated, walks over to the bed, sits down, and opens the drawer of her night table. She removes a stack of pamphlets from a variety of institutions in the area that she got from her father's doctor and Dr. Rivers's group sessions. She didn't honestly believe that she would ever have to resort to this—that is, until this very moment. She picks up the phone, dials the number, and waits for somebody to answer.

"Hello, Green Manor."

Chapter 8
Halloween 2008
6:00 a.m.

It is six o'clock in the morning, and Kathryn hasn't slept much. The sun has started to come up, and she's just lying in bed, lost in her thoughts as she stares at the ceiling. Rob is sound asleep next to her. Her thoughts are of the impending day and the events that have taken place over the past seven years. Suddenly, there is a knock at the door.

The door opens. Bobby, who is now twelve years old, walks in wearing an Iron Man Halloween mask on top of his head. He quietly but anxiously says, "Mom, Grandpa is picking the Thompsons' flowers again!

The Thompsons live next door, and Grandpa has picked flowers from their garden in the past. They were angry then, and there's no doubt they'll be angry again.

"Jesus, what time is it?" Rob asks in a sleepy voice.

"It's about six. Go back to sleep," Kathryn says to Rob. At this point, Bobby pulls his mask down over his face and jumps onto the bed. Although Rob pretends to be upset, he apparently accepts that his rest is over. He and Bobby begin to play on the bed as Kathryn hears Grandpa's voice as he comes down the hall.

"We three kings of Orient are," he sings, "bearing gifts we travel afar, field and fountain, moor and mountain, following yonder star. Oh, star of wonder, star of light, star with royal beauty bright, westward leading, still proceeding, guide us to thy perfect light."

Grandpa appears in the doorway dressed in street clothes over which he is wearing a bathrobe. As he approaches the bed, he extends an armful of flowers to her. He's definitely been into the Thompsons' flowers again, she thinks, and from the looks of it, he cleaned them out.

"Merry Christmas!" he chimes cheerily.

"Grandpa, it's Halloween," says Bobby as he removes the mask from his head, "not Christmas!"

Kathryn sits up, pulls back the comforter, and gets out of bed. She accepts the flowers and shushes him and Bobby in a semiserious way because she knows Rob won't want to get out of bed just yet. In a quiet voice, Kathryn thanks her father for the flowers.

"They're beautiful dad," she whispers. "But you know you shouldn't …"

"But this time," he interrupts her, "I did wear a coat!"

"Yeah, well anyway, now that we're all up, let's get you guys some breakfast."

Bobby starts calling out his order. "I want pancakes and cereal with bananas and …"

Kathryn shushes him and tells him to take his grandfather to the kitchen.

"I'll be right there, and keep your voices down, okay?"

As Grandpa and Bobby leave the room, Kathryn closes the door behind them. With a troubled look on her face, she turns back toward her husband.

"Do you think that he knows he's leaving today?" she asks.

"Kathryn, you know we decided ..." Rob cuts himself off, and then his tone becomes more compassionate. "Honey, he's going to be better off there. You've been so great with him. I mean, how many daughters would quit their job to care for their dad? But it's just too much to handle now."

"I know," she says. "I know. You're right."

Kathryn looks down for a moment at the flowers in her hand. A million images flood her mind as she thinks of all that her family has been through in the past seven years. Then, she turns and leaves the bedroom.

Chapter 9
Halloween 2008
7:45 a.m.

The time displayed on the wall clock in the kitchen reads 7:45 a.m. The family has just finished breakfast. Kathryn is still dressed in her pajamas and bathrobe, and she is clearing the table. Rob, wearing his work clothes, is reading the newspaper and finishing his coffee. Bobby is dressed and ready for school. He is at the counter fighting with his grandfather, who has since doffed his bathrobe, about how they should carve the pumpkin.

Kathryn wants to get the day's plans straight in her head, so she starts by questioning Bobby. After all, Halloween is, generally speaking, a holiday geared toward kids. There is a parade at Bobby's school, so he has to bring his costume with him. Then around seven o'clock, Bobby is supposed to be at the Whites' house. The plan is for the kids to get together and go trick-or-treating after they've all had dinner. Bobby's friend Steven lives in a safe neighborhood, and his family volunteered to take responsibility for Halloween this year.

As she visualizes the day's events in her head, Kathryn realizes that today is going to be very hectic. She still has so much packing to do, Bobby has school, then they have to take Grandpa to Green Manor, they have to have dinner, and then finally they have to get Bobby over to the Whites' house.

"Go finish getting ready for school," she says to Bobby, "and be careful with your costume. We aren't going to have much time when we get back from the home before we'll have to leave for Steven's."

"But Mom," he says as he continues to carve the pumpkin, "I don't want to go with you to take Grandpa."

"Bobby, get moving right now," Kathryn demands.

Bobby ignores his mother and continues to carve the pumpkin. Kathryn walks over to her son and removes the knife from his hand. Bobby whines, "Mooooom!" as he leaves the room to finish getting ready for school.

Through all of this Rob has not spoken a word. Now, he is leaning back in his chair and playing with the refrigerator magnets. Somebody had spelled out "Happy Halloween," and Rob is dismantling the word "Halloween." Although it doesn't appear that Rob is listening or really cares about what is going on with his family today, she knows he is and does.

"Honey," he says, "are we going to be able to make it back by seven? I really can't leave work till five, and …"

"Rob," Kathryn interrupts, "I want to leave here at five. Can't you get back sooner?"

"Why do you want to leave at five? We don't have to be at the home until six, right? So as long as I'm back by …"

"Yeah, but I don't want to take a chance that we get stuck in traffic," Kathryn interrupts again.

"All right," Rob concedes, "I'll be back by five at the latest, okay?"

"Thank you, dear." she says. "It's just …"

"I know, I know," interjects Rob sympathetically.

"I have to tell you, Rob," Kathryn says, "after the past several months of this, when I finally go back to work, it will be like a vacation."

Rob gets up from his chair at the table and walks over to his wife. He puts his arms around her and holds her for what seems to be an eternity. Meanwhile, Grandpa looks into space completely indifferent to the conversation that just took place.

Chapter 10
Halloween 2008
11:00 a.m.

Almost all of the preparations have been completed for Grandpa's move, but Kathryn did leave a few things for today. She has been following the advice of the doctors and nurses at Green Manor. She has taken a lot of her father's belongings to the home already, but she was told to hold off on packing the things he uses every day until as late as possible. That way he wouldn't be upset to find them missing.

In the early stages of dementia, Grandpa was convinced that his things were being stolen. It was at this point that the family doctor diagnosed the dementia that would lead to Alzheimer's disease. Although Kathryn and Rob knew something wasn't right and suspected Alzheimer's, it wasn't until the doctor mentioned the disease that it felt real.

The doctor had pontificated that Grandpa's paranoia would likely lead him to begin hiding his stuff. As it turned out, the doctor was correct, and a big topic of dinner conversation was often the location of her father's CDs. Her father was convinced that somebody was stealing them, so he would hide them. Then, when they weren't where he used to keep them, he would conclude that they had been stolen. The cycle was true not only for his CDs, but also for clothes, shoes, money, jewelry—basically anything and everything.

So knowing what she went through back then, Kathryn understood the frustration that her father would no doubt feel if, in fact, his belongings were to be removed. She wanted him to be as comfortable and at ease as possible in his last few days at the house. Besides, it was just as hard for her to remove them.

Today, however, the moment of truth has arrived. With a suitcase in one hand and a couple of boxes in the other, Kathryn enters her father's room to pack his remaining possessions. Her father isn't far behind her, and as she begins placing things in the boxes, he starts to hand her things to pack. Still, she thinks that he must be a bit rattled and is probably aware that something different and strange is happening today.

Kathryn goes over to the closet and takes out another suitcase. As she carries it across the room, she realizes that there is something inside. Perhaps her father was aware that he was moving. Maybe he started packing his own bags. She sets the case down and opens it. Inside she finds a bunch of flowers and a pile of dirt.

"What is all this stuff?" she asks. "Oh, Dad, these are more of the Thompsons' flowers. You were quite busy this morning."

"Why are you getting rid of me?" Grandpa asks, concerned. "I didn't mean to be bad; I promise I won't do it again."

Kathryn now sees the sadness in her father's eyes. She can tell by the tone of his voice that he is scared—almost terrified.

"Dad, I know it's scary," she says, trying to comfort him. "But there really is nothing to worry about. You haven't done anything wrong."

"You're not going to punish me, are you?"

"No, no, no, of course not. Everything is going to be okay; you just need to be in a place where they can take good care of you."

Grandpa appears satisfied, but perhaps more from the tone of her voice than by what she is saying. She knows that he no longer sees the events that are taking place as harmful. She has become quite adept at comforting him with her voice. It's by no means a science, but she has made it work for her on occasion.

Grandpa walks over to the closet, rattles around for a minute, and then emerges with a handful of hangers. He hands them to his daughter to pack.

"You don't need to take these, Dad," she says. "They have hangers there for you to use."

"They didn't have them in Hawaii!" he says emphatically.

Kathryn stops packing the bag and looks up at her father. She is a bit confused now that he is remembering this.

"Are you talking about your honeymoon?" she asks.

"Sure, don't you remember we didn't have anything to hang our clothes on?"

"What do you mean, Dad?" Kathryn asks, smiling. "I wasn't with you in Hawaii. You and Mom went there before I was born. You went there right after you were married. I'm your daughter, Dad."

"So you must have met us there, because I remember you were in the car when we drove from the airport ..."

"No, no, Dad. You were with Mom. Remember Mom? Laura. You two had just gotten married."

Kathryn goes over to the dresser and removes a picture frame from a drawer. She hands her father the photo and points at the picture of her mother.

"Her. Remember her? That's Mom, Laura Jean Rayne!"

Her father looks very frustrated and confused, but Kathryn persists. "That's who you were with. Not me. I'm your daughter. I'm Kathryn, not Laura."

Kathryn suddenly realizes that her father is getting frightened. She quickly puts the photograph down and places her arms around him. He seems to be on the verge of tears as Kathryn again shifts to a more soothing tone and starts to console her father, reassuring him that everything will be okay.

"I'm sorry, Dad. I didn't mean to upset you," she says while rocking him back and forth as if he were a child.

"If I leave, how will she get out?" he begs. "I can't help her. She needs me. I can't go."

"Who, Dad? Who needs help?"

"Laura. She's upstairs, and she needs me. She calls for me to help. I try to help her, but she's trapped up there. She needs me. I can't go."

Grandpa is now shaking, incoherent, and weeping. Kathryn just holds him. She knows that she set him off, but she also knows that she doesn't have the resources to care for him. She loves her father so much, and it is the most difficult thing for her not to be recognized by him as his daughter.

Chapter 11
Halloween 2008
12:30 p.m.

Kathryn prepares lunch for her father around midday—tomato soup and grilled cheese sandwiches served with potato chips, just the way he likes it. Her father eats the meal very slowly and methodically, which is his normal practice. The two of them do not generally tend to talk too much at lunch, although she likes to believe that her father enjoys the time together as much as she does. After he is finished, Grandpa gets up from the table and goes to the living room. It is his custom to watch a bit of television after he eats.

Kathryn clears the table and washes the dishes. When she is finished, she follows her father into the living room. She's not big into early afternoon TV, but she likes to use the time to read. She sits down in the chair in the corner of the room, and it's not long before she hears her father softly snoring. About fifteen minutes go by when the phone rings.

"Hello," Kathryn says into the phone after picking it up on the first ring.

"Hi, Kathryn, it's Christine," says the voice on the other end of the line. Kathryn and Christine have been friends for a long time. Not only was Christine the maid of honor at Kathryn's wedding, she is also Bobby's godmother.

"Oh, hi, Christine. How are you?" Kathryn says.

"I'm well. How are things over there today?"

"Pretty good, considering. He was picking the Thompsons' flowers again this morning, and he thinks it's Christmas. But same old, same old, right?"

"Does your dad know that he's moving, or how are you handling that?"

"Um, well, he knows something is different about today, I'm sure. Between Bobby's excitement and dressing up for Halloween, and me packing his clothes, I think he realizes that we're going somewhere. But he doesn't understand where, I don't think."

"I know that this has been tough on you, Kathryn. I don't know how you've managed to keep it together this long. Are you holding up okay?" Christine asks.

"I'm holding together very well, surprisingly. I've struggled with this decision for a long time, but that support group that I've been going to really has helped me to put things into perspective," Kathryn says.

"Well, you've certainly found him a great place to live. From what I can tell, Green Manor is a fantastic environment."

"Yeah, I mean I am absolutely sure that I'm doing what has to be done. He needs constant care now, and I can't, even with Rob's help, give him the kind of care he needs."

"Honestly, Kathryn, I don't think I could have done what you've done," Christine says. "You've given so much of yourself to take care of him. I imagine it's been tough on everybody over there, but you especially. I really admire your resolve, and I applaud you for having the strength to make such a difficult decision."

"Well, part of it really is selfish; I'd be lying if I denied it. But I have a life to live, and I tell you, Christine. I am so excited to be going back to work, if for no other reason than to get out of this house and interact with everyday, normal people again."

"Hey! What am I chopped liver?" Christine retorts with a chuckle.

"No, of course not. You've been really great. But you know what I mean. It hasn't been easy."

As Kathryn say this, her father wakes up. He seems disoriented, and he yells out, "Mommmmmmmmy!"

"Sorry, Christine, I have to go. Thank you so much, and I'll give you a call in the next couple of days," Kathryn says.

She goes over to her father and puts her arms around him.

"Dad, I'm here. I'm here, Dad," she says in a calming voice while rocking him back and forth. "Everything is okay,

Dad." Her father settles down and seems to get his bearings back again.

Chapter 12
Halloween 2008
2:00 p.m.

Grandpa is sitting on the bed in his room, staring off into space. It's impossible to know what he is thinking; perhaps he has no thoughts. Maybe he is in a sort of meditative trance, lost in a world of simple things—the lights, the sounds, the everyday ambiance that most people take for granted.

Kathryn walks into the room and begins looking for her father's pillbox. He insists on taking care of it himself. Of course, Kathryn takes care of all his prescription medication for him, but he doesn't know that. The pillbox he manages contains vitamins. The vitamin E, however, is important for him to take, especially in light of all the news that has emerged recently about the positive effect it has for Alzheimer's patients.

As she is looking around the room for the pills, she asks him if he has taken them yet today. He, of course, replies in the affirmative. When she finally finds the box, she knows that, in fact, he has not yet taken the pills in the Friday section.

"Oh, Dad, you did not take them," she says. "They're right here."

"There they are," he replies as he picks his nose.

"Here, Dad, you need to take these. They're gonna make you feel better."

"No! I don't want those."

"All right, Dad, that's okay. How about a drink? Are you thirsty?" Grandpa nods, and Kathryn goes off to the kitchen to concoct an elixir. She mashes up the pills and mixes them into a glass of juice. When she's finished, she returns to her father's room and hands him the glass. He accepts the glass and takes a sip. As soon as the liquid hits his tongue, Grandpa spits it out dramatically onto the floor.

"Why are you making me drink this?" he demands. "It's awful."

"Oh, stop being so melodramatic," says Kathryn. "It's not that bad."

"Well, I'll have nothing to do with your tricks. If you want to treat me like a child, then maybe I'll act like one."

"That's fine, Dad, but one way or another you will take your medicine."

"Might I remind you," he says angrily, "that I am a grown man. In fact, I'm your father. I raised you, and I think that you owe me a modicum of respect. I didn't put sweat, blood, and tears into raising a rude, pushy, overbearing daughter. And another thing young lady …"

"Oh, get off your high horse. Don't take the pills, take the pills, do whatever you want. I'm sorry I cared," she says as she leaves the room.

As she leaves, she hears him say under his breath, "Good." He then drinks the rest of the juice.

Chapter 13
Halloween 2008
4:45 p.m.

Although Kathryn seemed to have everything under control this morning, by late afternoon everything is whirling out of control. Rob should be home anytime now. Bobby has returned home from school with a torn costume. So Kathryn is in the Music Room sewing it while Grandpa sits in there with her, not doing much of anything. Bobby walks into the room carrying a Jonathon Rayne performance poster.

"Let's put this one over here, Grandpa!" he says excitedly.

"Not now, Bobby," Kathryn scolds. "This is still Grandpa's room."

"But look, Mom, I have it all figured out. We can put the computer over here, and all the games on the shelf, and right here by the pictures, I'll put the flute Grandpa gave me."

Bobby is speaking with such enthusiasm that his grandfather gets caught up in the excitement. It's almost as if this nearly eighty-year-old man is a kid playing a game.

"What do you think, Grandpa?" Bobby asks. "A dartboard over here?"

"Hey, hey, hey, Bobby, come on; we can do all that later," says his mother.

Bobby playfully punches his grandfather in the arm, and Grandpa in turn grabs Bobby and proceeds to give him a noogie. The two of them are wrestling like a couple of young brothers.

"That's enough, you two!" Kathryn says as Rob walks into the room.

"You guys about ready to go?" he asks.

Kathryn has finished sewing the costume, and she stands up to give Rob a hug.

"Actually honey," she says, "I've been thinking. Maybe I'll just take Dad on my own."

"We can all go. I'm sure we can make it back on time."

"I know, Rob, and I appreciate your support, but I think I want to be alone with him."

"Are you sure, Kathryn?"

"Yeah, you take Bobby out to get some dinner and then take him over to the Whites."

"Okay, no problem. I'll see you later then." Rob kisses his wife and then calls out to his son, "Hey, Bobbo, it's you and me for dinner tonight!"

"Oh, and Rob I fixed his costume, but you'll just need to reattach the rubber band to his mask. It came apart at school.

Just use some tape or something. I'm sure Mrs. White will have something."

"Will do. All right, let's go, Bobby. Make sure you have all your stuff."

Bobby picks up his costume and heads for the door. Grandpa is also walking toward the door. As they both are about to pass Kathryn, she grabs them each by their wrists. Almost as if Grandpa is her second child, she says, "And make sure these hands are clean."

As she says this, holding her father's hand, she realizes that this may be the last time she will be standing with him in this room—this room filled with so many memories and memorabilia from his life. She is overcome with sadness and engulfed in nostalgia. She lets Bobby go, and he is off to dinner with his father.

Meanwhile, she holds a bit tighter to her father's hand and then embraces him in a hug.

Chapter 14
Halloween 2008
6:00 p.m.

They pull up to the driveway of the Green Manor nursing home after about forty minutes in the car. The driveway is about a quarter of a mile long, and at the end of it is the entrance to the main building. There is a small parking lot in front of the building and a larger one on the side.

The front of the building is like a hotel or hospital. She can pull right up to the main entrance under an overhang. The area is meant for drop-offs and pickups—occasionally by ambulances. However, the staff at Green Manor told her to park there to make it easier to bring in her father and his things.

The place is beautifully kept with grass everywhere and neatly trimmed bushes. Kathryn had seen the place in the summer when she first came to check out the facility and staff. At that time, the flowers were in bloom, and it was magnificent. They even have benches scattered throughout the grounds; it really is a gorgeous place. And of course, it's currently all done up for the holiday, complete with dried corn stalks and jack-o'-lanterns out front.

Most important, though, is that everybody on the staff, especially the head of patient care, Nurse Conway, seems to be very helpful and accommodating. The grounds, facility, staff, and residents all seem perfect, which contributes to putting Kathryn's mind at ease.

Kathryn gets out of the car and walks over to the passenger's side where her father is. He is getting out of the car as she approaches, and she takes his hand as she closes the door. The two of them walk arm and arm up the steps to the main entrance.

Once inside, they check in at the reception desk. Kathryn is given a visitors badge and told that somebody will go out and get her father's bags. As Kathryn hands her car keys to the lady behind the desk, she sees Nurse Conway walking down the hall toward her. "What service!" Kathryn thinks to herself.

"Hello, Mrs. Wilder and Mr. Rayne!" Nurse Conway greets them both with warmth and enthusiasm. The three of them begin walking down the hall to Grandpa's new room. Nurse Conway introduces them to almost every person they pass along the way.

When they arrive at Grandpa's room, they see that all of the things that Kathryn had brought before were laid out. It isn't more than a few minutes before the bags and boxes from the car are brought in by a young orderly.

"I'll leave you two to say good-bye," Nurse Conway says to Kathryn. "Oh, and before I forget, there are a couple more papers for you to sign. So please stop by the front desk on your way out."

Then Nurse Conway turns to Grandpa and says to him, "I'll be back in a few minutes to introduce you to the rest of your neighbors, and then we'll go down to dinner." As she leaves the room, she turns to him, winks, and says, "You're gonna break a lot of hearts!"

Kathryn begins unpacking her father's things and putting them away.

"Did she mean we're going to eat here?" Grandpa asks. "Or are we going to get something to eat on the train?"

"No, no, Dad. This isn't the train station. This is Green Manor, your new home."

"Well, I've never lived in a train station before," says Grandpa incredulously.

"Of course not," Kathryn says simply.

When Kathryn finishes unpacking the rest of her father's things, she walks over to him and begins to straighten his clothes.

"You sure are a handsome devil," she says.

He just smiles at her in an apathetic sort of way. Kathryn is sad, and the emotion of the situation is catching up to her.

"It's time to say good-bye, Dad. I love you very much, and I'll be back in a couple of days, okay?"

"Okay," he says.

Kathryn wraps her arms around her father and squeezes him tight. Then she kisses him on the forehead as a tear falls down her cheek. She turns to leave the room, and as she reaches the door, she turns back to her father and says, "Good-bye, Dad, you old heartbreaker!"

Grandpa sits on the bed as Kathryn turns to leave. The only sound she hears is that of her own footsteps as she walks slowly down the hall.